Living Proof

A Cancer-Free Miracle

Living Proof

A Cancer-Free Miracle

Courage and Collaboration
Faith and Love

Irungu Adeyemi

Adeyemi Books

Adeyemi Books™
Temecula, California
www.AdeyemiBooks.com

10 9 8 7 6 5 4 3 2
First Edition Published 2011
Printed in the United States of America

Published in collaboration with
Grassroots Publishing Group

ISBN-10: 0-9794805-4-X
ISBN-13: 978-0-9794805-4-6
Library of Congress Control Number: 2011927597

Image of "Fruit in Bowl" on p. 57 by Alem Roberts
Cover & book design by CenterPointe Media
www.CenterPointeMedia.com

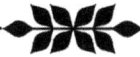

Miracles blossom

in the soil of

effort,

attitude,

and faith.

DEDICATION

I dedicate this book to
God, the Almighty
My wife, Marilyn
My children and grandchildren

I also dedicate this book to
My parents, Teena and Porter, and
My wife's parents,
Julia and James, Sr.

Acknowledgments

God smiles down on those who teach children. In order to support my continued success as a teacher, He placed specific individuals in my life who provided me the courage, strength, and motivation I needed to be effective and focused during my battle with cancer. I would like to thank and recognize the following people:

My wife, Marilyn J. Adeyemi, whom I love with all my heart. When you called me your "hero," you inspired me to fight for my life. Thank you for being by my side every step of the way. My three children—Alem, Telinda, and Tony—for your love and support. I hope that my victory over cancer inspires you to never give up ... despite the odds against you.

Thomas Sweet, M.D. (oncologist), for your positive attitude and your passion for fighting for your patients ... despite their prognoses and the odds against them.

Bill and Ernestine Martin for your prayers and encouragement, and for your nutritional drink recipe that enhanced my immune system; your kindness and friendship remain forever close to my heart. Elias and Maryhelen Garcia, for your prayers and for supplying me with a juicer to blend my nutritional juice drink; your thoughtfulness and support will be remembered always. Margaret Villalobos, for your prayers and friendship during a time when my family and I needed to hear encouraging words.

Dr. George Cameron, for your sensitivity in pointing out that technology has come a long way and I would be just fine; your caring words meant so much to me. Frankie Escobeto, my supervisor, for your kindness and support during a very difficult time in my life; you will never know the depth of my appreciation for your encouragement and friendship. My colleagues at John A. Otis School, for cheering me on and for offering many, many prayers for me and my family; each one of you helped encourage and motivate me. My colleagues at the National School District/Sweetwater U.H.S.D (Regional Occupational Program), for your outpouring of compassion, prayers, and support; you will remain in my heart forever. The National School District Board members and Teachers' Association, for all your prayers and support.

My daughter, Alem Roberts, for her beautiful interior art.

To all the angels who appeared along the way, I thank you for keeping me positive during difficult times.

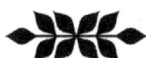

Contents

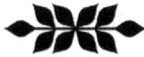

Foreword

Reflecting on my twenty-plus years of experience in the education field, I find myself pondering the many influences and events that led me to my current position of leading the largest elementary school district in the state of California. I was blessed to have worked with outstanding leaders in the field, along with amazing teachers who transformed young lives and families. Yet one individual teacher will always stand out as probably the most courageous and dedicated person I have ever known—Mr. Irungu Adeyemi.

Samuel Johnson defined courage as the greatest of all virtues, because unless a man has that virtue, he has no security for preserving any other. Irungu personified this virtue during my four years as principal at John A. Otis Elementary School, a school located in National City a few miles south

of San Diego and about ten miles north of the U.S.-
Mexico border. It was a school that many saw as
challenging since the neighborhood had the highest
gang ratio in the nation and over 90 percent of the
population lived below the poverty line. However,
Mr. Adeyemi perceived this community using another lens, and what he saw was a beautiful hamlet
filled with hope and a hunger for knowledge.

Irungu Adeyemi dedicated his entire profes-
sional career, over thirty years, to lay the founda-
tion for many students who later would come
back to his sixth-grade classroom to share their
accomplishments of being accepted into prestigious
universities, and to share their gratitude for the
instrumental part he played in their journey to a
better life. Like other many heroes of the past, his
great sacrifices came with a cost that almost took
his life.

Even though Irungu could have worked a few
miles from home in his upper middle class neighborhood in Temecula, he traveled ninety minutes each
way to one of the most dangerous school districts in
California. He accumulated close to a year of sick
leave because his attendance was impeccable and
he never missed work, until the immemorial day
he shared the diagnosis that he had contracted a
fatal condition. Mr. Adeyemi had an advanced state
of lung cancer and was given little hope of recovery.

The following account will define the essence of
the man who struggled through a debilitating ill-

ness that shook the fabric of our community and his family. It gives us hope and courage that it is possible to move mountains, and it gives us the fight to struggle with every inch of our fiber. Mr. Irungu Adeyemi is truly an inspiration to every person who dares to be called a teacher.

Francisco Escobedo, Ed.D.
Superintendent
Chula Vista Elementary School District
Chula Vista, California

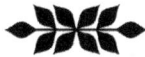

Preface

I wrote this book to help two distinct populations: (1) people who are facing their own battles with cancer, and (2) people who are helping their loved ones through a difficult health challenge. This book is meant to give you hope and inspire you *never* to give up. Yes, life has changed for you—you are now a patient or a caretaker—but that doesn't mean that life is over. Actually, when you are struggling with illness, some things become clearer than ever. Life and health begin to look like the gifts they are, gifts that should have been cherished all along. Often humans take things such as health for granted, but that mindset changes when you are facing cancer head on.

I am living proof that *miracles do happen.* Thirteen years ago I faced a three-month death sentence. I knew I had to decide quickly how I was going to handle the news and what I was going to do with it, so I asked myself, "Do I lay down and give in, or do I stand up and fight?"

I chose to stand up and fight, and I pray that you choose to do the same. In order to receive God's blessings, you must partner with God. You must do the work and take the steps necessary to heal yourself. God will stand with you if you let him in, and his angels will appear in different colors, shapes, and forms along the way. I believe God's love increases during times of illness as he readily shares your experience with you. Open your heart to receive God's blessings. If you don't yet know God, seek him out. He will bless you for your efforts.

I pray that my words will inspire you and your loved ones to believe, as I do, that *miracles do happen* and they come from a merciful God who partners with you and eternally loves you.

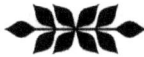

CHAPTER ONE
The New School Year

When the new school year began, I was full of enthusiasm, which is a wonderful way for a teacher to start the school year. As a matter of fact, my students were just as eager as I was. They stood before me wearing brand new uniforms, shoes, and smiles. Feeling the positive vibrations emanate from a group of children who are energized to start the school year is one of the most satisfying feelings a teacher can experience. This was their last year before entering junior high, so "Let's get rolling" was the general consensus between most of the sixth graders and their new teachers.

I prided myself on being a teacher whom students hoped to get, and the one that parents requested. Teaching was very important to me. I came out of an era and educational system in which many of the teachers wrote the assignments on the

blackboard with chalk and then sat at their desks
for the rest of the day. Because of my educational
experience, I felt it was not only my job to prepare
my students for the future, but also my duty. Therefore, I accepted a challenge: to be one of the best
and most effective teachers my students would ever
have in their lifetimes.

I had another reason, a personal reason, to feel
enthusiastic. During a recent medical checkup for
a persistent cough, it was determined that I might
be experiencing allergy symptoms instead of something more serious. Up to that point, I hadn't even
considered the big "C," but I knew that something
was wrong. I had never had a cough such as that
before. In fact, I hardly ever caught colds.

Soon we were several weeks into the school
year; I was working hard and maintaining my
enthusiasm. I did not want anything to diminish or
interrupt the energy of the new school year.

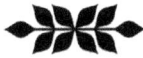

CHAPTER TWO

Your Doctor Would Like to See You

With thoughts of my medical condition running through the back of my mind, I felt that it would be prudent to inform my principal that I was waiting for test results concerning a cough that had persisted for sometime now. My principal, being a supportive person, provided me with words of encouragement. "Everything will work out just fine," he said as he patted me on the shoulder. To this day he doesn't know how reassuring it was to hear those encouraging words and how deeply I appreciated them then and continue to appreciate them now.

A week or so later, shortly after recess, my principal came into my classroom. He said, "Excuse me, Mr. Adeyemi. There is a phone call for you at the office. It's your doctor's office calling."

We didn't have telephones in our classrooms back then. Instead, we used intercoms to communicate with the office. Judging by the sound of my principal's voice and his body language, I could tell that the news I was about to hear wasn't going to be good. Perhaps the person he spoke to had concern in his or her voice. My principal motioned toward the main building and said, "I'll take over your class while you take your call."

The walk to the main office took forever. When I got there, I heard myself saying, "Hello. This is Irungu Adeyemi speaking."

The voice on the other side said, "Yes, Mr. Adeyemi. Your doctor would like you to stop by this evening to take some X-rays. Your results are negative for allergies. It is important that you keep the appointment this evening. You can go directly to the X-ray area. They have a stat request waiting for you. Will you be able to keep this appointment?"

Immediately I answered, "Yes. I'll stop by on my way home. Thank you."

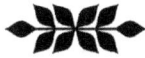

CHAPTER THREE

X-Rays

The walk back to my classroom was much quicker than the walk to the office to answer the phone. Because I didn't want to dwell on what I was going to face that evening, I felt an urgency to be back in the classroom teaching.

I thanked my principal for his concern and informed him that the previous tests showed up negative for allergies, and I had to go in for X-rays that evening. My principal insisted that I take off the rest of the afternoon. He said, "I'll get someone in here for you. You have to take care of yourself."

I thanked him, but I insisted that I would rather finish out the day. He agreed with me because by now my students were trying to figure out why the principal was asking me to take off the rest of the afternoon. I appreciated the principal's sensitivity. He truly was a caring people-person.

I decided not to bother my wife with the news

straight away. I knew that she would be greatly
concerned that I had to take X-rays that evening.
She was also a teacher. By informing her later, I
avoided disrupting her time with her students.
The afternoon did not pass fast enough for me.
Finally, I had to tell my wife about the X-rays. I
knew this was not something she was going to want
to hear, and by now it was starting to weigh heavily
on my mind, as well.

As I entered my wife's classroom, she sensed
that something was not right. "What's wrong?" she
asked with concern in her voice.

I informed her that I received my test results earlier that day, and they found no signs of allergies
causing my cough. "I have been asked to stop by on
the way home to take X-rays."

I knew I had to stay positive at this point because I had to stay strong for my wife. "Don't worry.
Everything will be just fine," I whispered into her
ear as I held her in my arms. The drive to the medical center seemed to last forever, and forever my life
was about to change.

As I unbuttoned my shirt in the X-ray room,
I remember feeling dwarfed by the huge medical
apparatus that was filling the space. Did the technician ask me to keep my undershirt on or take it off?
While I was preoccupied with my ponderings about
what might be wrong with me, the technician's
instructions floated in and out of my ears. "Could it
be cancer?" I thought. Standing in the cold, sterile

X-ray room caused all sorts of thoughts to enter my mind. Suddenly my thinking was interrupted by a voice over the intercom that said, "You may keep your undershirt on."

Before I knew it, I was positioned to stand with my chest against the cold X-ray panel. My chin rested in a chin rest, and my shoulders were pinned against the panel. The proper positioning was important to ensure a perfect X-ray.

From behind a glass partition I heard, "Take a deep breath ... hold ... now breathe out."

Then I was asked to stand perpendicular to the panel. "Hold your arms above your head," the technician requested politely while she scooted me closer to the panel to prepare for a different view of my lungs. Once again, the voice behind the thick glass requested, "Now, take a deep breath ... hold ... breathe out."

At this point I sent a prayer to God asking for protection from whatever I might be facing. "Just let it not be cancer," I whispered to myself.

As I tried to collect myself, the voice behind the glass echoed, "You may get dressed."

As my wife and I started to leave the lab area, we heard a voice behind us saying, "Don't leave without seeing your doctor this evening." The X-ray technician who just took the X-rays had noticeable concern in her voice.

Immediately I asked, "Is there a problem?"

She replied, "Just try to see your doctor before

you leave this evening."

I tried not to think the worst, but judging from the technician's persistence and the frightened expression that swept across my wife's face, I knew something serious was going on.

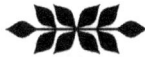

CHAPTER FOUR

I'm Afraid You Have Cancer

I met with my doctor. I'm sure some of the most dreaded words in any language are, "I'm afraid you have cancer." I can't say that I had an immediate panic reaction to what he just told me. I felt something more like a general numbness as I tried to interpret his words. After all, several months ago I had been examined by a nurse practitioner who thought my cough was the result of an allergic reaction. Now I was being confronted with a diagnosis of lung cancer.

As I gave my doctor my undivided attention, my numbness began to fade. Both my wife and I sat motionless as the doctor simultaneously reached for a piece of paper on his desk and a pen from his jacket pocket. He placed the paper in front of my wife and me and began to draw what appeared to be a lung.

As the pen traveled in circles that pinpointed

where the tumors were located, my doctor said in a sturdy and reassuring voice, "This is the affected area." At this point it became very clear that I had a medical problem. This was not a biology lesson that I was teaching to my students. This was a diagnosis of malignant tumors (non-small cell) that were located over a portion of my upper left lung.

The doctor was being straight up with me during his presentation, which gave me some comfort while I was struggling to process the information he was delivering about my diagnosis. Yet it was a time and space that was difficult to describe because I couldn't imagine what the doctor was telling me—that I had cancer. If there were ever a time I felt blindsided, this was it. Because I lived a healthy lifestyle, I asked myself, "How could *I* come down with cancer ... at the *beginning* of the school year?"

I thought to myself, "Is this a bad dream, or is this a moment in reality that thousands of people face each and every day?"

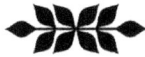

CHAPTER FIVE

Reviewing My Life

My doctor continued in a steady voice, the same voice that moments earlier said, "I'm afraid you have lung cancer." Now the voice was saying, "I can't see how surgery can be an option for you because the tumors are located in the upper areas of your lung. If the tumors were located on the lower lobe, then surgery would be an option." It appeared that surgery was not a viable alternative in my case.

It was apparent that the doctor had studied my X-rays before my wife and I got to his office. In his mind he knew it was over for me, but he proceeded to do what he had to do—make his presentation. He pointed out that I had a non-small-cell form of cancer, most likely environmental and not the result of smoking. That was encouraging to me because I had stopped smoking about fifteen years earlier in order to do what I could to head off a day like this. I thought, "At least I am not responsible for my own demise." The idea of taking care of myself popped up front and center at that moment. Nevertheless, I still had come down with cancer.

I stared straight ahead at the piece of paper that had, in mere moments, revealed my destiny. The words "I can't see how surgery can be an option here" became clearer to me. As I held my wife's hand, I felt the emotional stress she was experiencing. Her anxiety hurt me more than being told that I had cancer and was facing imminent death.

At this point my mind became remarkably keen. Instantaneously, I reviewed my life as if it were a movie flashing through my mind. The review happened so swiftly that I didn't even have time to think. Yet, at the same time, everything seemed to be moving in slow motion.

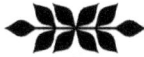

CHAPTER SIX
I Was Not Afraid

Despite experiencing the flashback of my entire life, I felt a calmness I cannot explain as I sat with my doctor and my terrified wife. In an attempt to understand the flashback with some sense of clarity, I can say that it summed up everything I had experienced in my life. Most important, it highlighted how I treated others and how I responded to the way others treated me. In essence, the flashback represented the kind of person I had become as a result of my own life experiences.

Flickers of life ran through the mind in a way that compares to an ember that bursts free from a burning log, or a spark that generates from static electricity. Embers and sparks die out as quickly as they are born—and so did my flashback. As a result of being told that I had terminal cancer, I felt myself being lifted to a place that, ultimately, every one of us will encounter. I was staring death in the face. But I was not afraid. I had a deep faith in God and a positive attitude. I knew that even though all the odds were stacked against me, it wasn't my time yet.

"I will schedule an appointment with a surgeon," my doctor said in a concerned voice that was nothing like the more reassuring voice he had used earlier when he first announced that I had cancer. Since my cancer was inoperable, he was sending me off to get the final word. I could tell that this was something he had trouble coming to terms with— sending me to a surgeon for inoperable tumors and a definitive prognosis. It had been easy and familiar for him to inform me that I had cancer, but now he had empathy in his voice as he handed me the sketch of my tumor-infected lung.

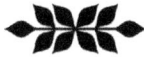

CHAPTER SEVEN
Asking God for a Miracle

I took the drawing from the doctor, thanked him, and prepared to leave with my wife for a weekend that would be full of unknowns. Actually, I don't remember in what manner my wife and I departed the medical center. Were we talking to each other? Did we notice the other people around us? Had I asked the doctor any questions while he was telling us that I had terminal lung cancer? Honestly, I can't remember anything except the feeling of knowing that I was facing something that no human being ever wants to face.

Even though my wife and I were not aware of anything outside of ourselves on the drive home, we arrived to our house safely. I remember standing in our walk-in closet and letting out a sigh—not a sigh of complaint or a sigh of "Why me?" but a sigh that conveyed that facing death is a humbling experience.

Throughout my life I routinely thanked God, regardless of where I was at any particular moment. Therefore, it was not difficult for me to ask God now to please come into my life and heal me. I felt I was in good standing with God, and I know that my peace of mind was coming directly from that belief.

The next step was to call my mother and give her the news. Because of her strong faith, I knew that she would have comforting words for me, and I was correct. I remember her advice, it was clear as day: "Put your dilemma into the hands of God, and you'll be healed." That was the moment I first realized the seriousness of what I was facing. In essence, my mother was advising me to let go of the steering wheel. She was telling me to take my situation to the altar and then step back. Stepping up to the altar felt right, but instead of stepping back, I chose to partner with God. It was not that I didn't trust Him to heal me without my help; it was, instead, that I was asking Him to perform a miracle. Did I merit such a blessing? Of course, I liked to think so, but in God's perspective, was I one of the people who deserved such a marvel? Did God hold me in such favor?

I decided to do whatever I could to help God help me. First, I went on the Internet to seek as much information as I could about lung cancer. I wanted to know what I was facing and if there was anything I could do to help God help me. After all, I was raised to believe that "God helps those who help themselves."

During my research I discovered that if surgery is possible, the patient's chances for survival are greatly enhanced. Furthermore, if patients receive chemotherapy and radiation treatments that eradicate their cancer tumors, their life expectancy could be extended five years. With this information in hand, I was determined to come up with a strategy to fight for my life.

First, I acknowledged that my wife needed me by her side. Next, I recognized that I wanted to survive for my family and my students. Further, I resolved to finish out the school year with my class. My family, my work, and my students weighed heavily on my mind.

Soon I received an appointment with a surgeon. Because I had been told by the throat-and-lung doctor that surgery would be out of the question in my case, I greeted this appointment with apprehension. But being a positive person who believes that prayers can be answered, I remained optimistic and looked forward to being informed that surgery would, after all, be a possibility in my case.

My wife and I prayed hard for surgery to be an option.

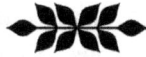

CHAPTER EIGHT

Appointment with My Surgeon

My appointment with my surgeon was not a positive one. It took me, literally, several years to reverse the damage caused by his attitude toward me and his manner while communicating with me. Medical doctors are given authority over the lives of their patients, and when they know there is nothing that can be done medically to improve a bad situation, they should, without hesitation, give their patients their utmost respect. This surgeon didn't know that God was going to perform a miracle on me. I didn't know it yet either. But no matter what my prognosis was, I should have been treated respectfully.

The surgeon told me that there wasn't anything that could be done to save my life. Surgery was out of the picture, he said. He plainly avoided making eye contact with me. In every way, his demeanor painted a clear picture of the seriousness of the situation I faced.

In a short while my appointment concluded. After my wife and I were already standing, the surgeon asked me if I had any questions. I didn't feel as if he had placed me in a position to comfortably question him. Instead, it appeared as if I was there for one reason only ... to receive my death sentence. Even though my appointment was a let's-hurry-up-and-get-it-over-with session, I decided that I wasn't going to leave without pointing out to the surgeon that I was going to do what I could to try to save my life.

"Yes, Doctor. I have a question. What do you think of vitamin supplements?" I asked this question with great confidence because vitamin supplements were one of the ways I chose to work with God to help myself. Immediately the surgeon told me that there wasn't any scientific evidence to support any benefit from taking supplements to fight cancer.

That was the first and last contact I had with my appointed surgeon. As he walked away, I asked, "How much time do I have?" He replied, "Ninety days to a year." Then he left.

I hope one day to show that surgeon that medical doctors should never give up on their patients ... because *miracles* do, without a doubt, happen. *I am living proof of it.*

After this startling appointment, I became determined to pray even harder and to continue my research. I resolved to read only information that was positive in nature and included specifics that could lead to a cure. I did not want to waste my time dwelling on information that could "take the wind out of my sail." I would be satisfied as long as I could keep the wind to my back until I reached "a port with a cure."

The cure rate for lung cancer is very low. As a result of the odds stacked against me, I visualized myself being in that small percentage of people who would be blessed with a cure. I knew in my heart that God would hear my prayers and intervene to heal me.

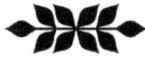

CHAPTER NINE
Supplements

The surgeon didn't know that I had God on my side. To him I was a statistic. I would have preferred him to show some empathy. It would have been nice to hear him say, "You know what? Chemotherapy or radiation might be a way to lick this cancer." I wanted and needed to hear a proposal that offered an option or words that alluded to a fighting chance. Some form of compassionate communication would have been encouraging. I was facing imminent death, and I would have benefited from hearing kind words.

On my own I started a vitamin regimen (see Appendix):
- vitamin C
- vitamin E
- selenium

Allegedly, these antioxidants are cancer cell destroyers. When patients are fighting for their lives and searching for the strength to stay positive—by believing that vitamins, or a placebo for that matter, are going to help them save their lives—how can any medical expert destroy their hopes?

I decided to take the surgeon's opinion with a grain of salt. I wasn't going to permit him to destroy my positive attitude. Nor should any of you let anyone destroy yours. You must stay positive. You must stand up to cancer. You cannot take it lying down.

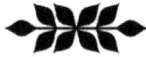

CHAPTER TEN
Prayers, Phone Calls, and Encouragement

By this time, and with my consent, most of my colleagues in my school district had been made aware of my lung cancer. Immediately prayers went up, and I was bombarded with phone calls from so many people who wished me the best in my fight with cancer. The staff at John Otis School, lead by a very special principal, were wonderful to me and my family. I'll never forget their many prayers, kindnesses, and encouragement.

In addition, the prayers and encouragement I received from my adult school class at the Regional Occupational Program, backed by my director and staff members, were also appreciated by me and my family during this time of uncertainty. I'll always cherish their support and thoughtfulness.

Also etched in my memory are the positive words my superintendent spoke to me: "Irungu, technology has come a long way. You'll do just fine in your treatments."

Each and every positive word, thought, and prayer that poured my way has been a blessing to me and my family. And I'm sure, regardless of your particular illness, that prayer and faith in the almighty God will help to provide a miracle for you and your family.

At this point I had no knowledge of what would become of me. I hoped that God would answer all of the prayers that had been sent to him on my behalf and that technology had come a long way, as Dr. Cameron, my district superintendent, had said.

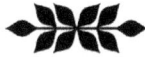

CHAPTER ELEVEN
Meeting with My Oncologist

S ince surgery was not an option for me, everything began to move swiftly. By now information was pouring in from every which way. One suggestion was that I try to get accepted by a popular oncologist who had been around for many years helping patients with their battles against cancer. When I was told that he had a long waiting list, I was disappointed. Well, at least I tried.

About a week later I was scheduled to meet my appointed oncologist. My wife and I waited anxiously in the reception area to meet the next important person to appear in our lives, the one who was going to join me, my wife, and God in my battle against terminal lung cancer. The wait was endless but was worth every moment.

When my wife and I were waiting in the examination room, we heard an enthusiastic knock on the door. A very young-looking doctor entered the room.

He eagerly stuck out his hand in greeting and said in a welcoming tone, "Hello. I am your oncologist." My wife and I were elated to have such a positive personality on our team. He was young *and* positive, and that was enough for me.

In unison my wife and I said, "Hello. Nice to meet you." The young doctor continued, "I am going to fight this cancer very aggressively, first with chemotherapy, then with radiation." His words were music to our ears. Now I had another fighter on my side: God, my oncologist, my wife and I ... and the angels who were still to come.

The moment I met my oncologist, I believed God brought him into my life to provide me with a special gift that was waiting for me at the end of this process. And I learned an important lesson, as well: A person's age makes no difference whatsoever. A positive attitude is what counts at a time like this.

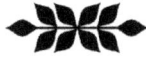

CHAPTER TWELVE
Information and Support

It wasn't long after meeting my oncologist that my youngest daughter, Alem Aisha, presented me with a book about how to stay positive while fighting cancer (see Appendix). It talked about being positive and creating mental images designed to fight the cancer that was attacking my healthy cells. The antioxidants in the supplements I took were now considered my warriors. This book was a very important tool in my battle; it helped me assist God with my healing process and prepared me to receive a miracle. My daughter knew I was a positive person already, and perhaps she felt that the book would build on my already upbeat character. She was right. It certainly did.

The *Bible* was the cornerstone of the faith I had in God's word. My wife and I began to travel 125 miles round trip to a church that we had noticed off the freeway during our workday commutes. This church was an excellent experience for both of us. We felt at home as we enjoyed their fellowship and the word of God.

God had always been in our home and our lives, despite the fact that we hadn't always had a physical building to worship in. The companionship and the devotion of this church were critical to us at this precarious time.

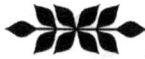

CHAPTER THIRTEEN
No Time to Pout

After meeting with my oncologist, my wife and I walked out of his office with information in hand on my first chemotherapy appointment. I was fired up with positive feelings about winning my battle with the most dreaded disease on the face of Earth. I know I am using the word "battle" repeatedly, but that's because it describes exactly what I was in—a battle for my life. Cancer is not something to take lightly. I was approaching stage four, which is very serious. I was losing more weight every day, and my tumors were inoperable. Yes, I was definitely battling for my life.

Shortly after my wife and I arrived home, she said to me, "Baby, you're my *hero*." Her words meant so much to me. Heroes do not stand on the sidelines and mope. On the contrary, they take care of business. I guess that's what my wife was seeing in me.

I must have impressed her with my attitude

because after we returned home she wanted to go out to our favorite Mexican food restaurant in downtown Temecula. Can you believe that? I was told I was dying of inoperable lung cancer, and she was calling me her hero and wanting to go out to eat. She and I understood that seeing the lighter side of a situation and having appreciation for what you have are important tools when you are fighting for your life.

Subsequently, my wife became my hero. She never gave me time to pout or feel sorry for myself. She knew that I was the type of person who, most likely, would not sit around and sulk, but she wasn't going to take any chances.

Another special gift came to me by the way of two wonderful friends, Bill and Ernestine Martin, who practice a nutritional lifestyle through their Seventh Day Adventist faith. Bill and Ernestine provided me with a juice recipe, a concoction of fruits and vegetables, intended to build up my immune system (see Appendix). A healthy immune system is critical when fighting illness, especially cancer. This gift from them will always be cherished by me and shared with others. The Martins had already shared it with many other people who were in the same or similar situation I was in.

Upon hearing that the Martins had given me a recipe consisting of antioxidant fruits and veg-etables, another bighearted family immediately offered my wife their brand new juicer so I could have my nutritional drink that same day. Elias and Maryhelen Garcia and their mother Margaret Villalobos will remain forever in my heart for their generosity.

Everything was falling into place: I had God, my wife, daughters, son, extended family, and so many other wonderful people doing everything they could to save my life.

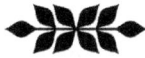

CHAPTER FOURTEEN
Chemotherapy

Chemotherapy introduced me to my new identity—cancer patient. Prior to that, I was an everyday family man, husband, father, and teacher who happened to come down with lung cancer.

Naturally, I felt apprehension before and during my very first chemo session. While I was in the waiting room anticipating my call for treatment, I didn't know what to expect. My wife and I sat quietly, as did everyone else in the room. I was sitting with about twenty other patients who were accompanied by spouses, friends, or parents. No one made eye contact with anyone else; however, there was plenty of empathy in the air. All of us were in the same boat. It didn't matter if we were young, old, black, white, or Latino. We all were fighting for our lives or the lives of our loved ones. I said a prayer for everyone who sat in that waiting room that day.

The only way we were going to win this battle was by the grace of God.

Finally, someone called me in to begin my chemotherapy session. To tell you the truth, everything went smoothly. I received the hookup—a long needle inserted into a vein on the backside of my hand along the wrist—with some apprehension. But I concentrated on the fact that I was taking my first step toward healing. That's the way I had to view my situation if I was going to be serious about winning my battle with cancer.

My wife, being a very practical person, realized that it was lunchtime. She asked the nurse if I could have lunch while I was receiving my chemo. The nurse said that lunch wouldn't be a problem, and she ordered me a meal. I thought that made sense until my oncologist happened by. "Mr. Adeyemi," he cried out, "you're going to have everyone in here throwing up." Of course he was joking, but the reason behind his words was serious. Nausea is the number one side effect of chemotherapy. If patients who experience this side effect are receiving treatment and watch someone else eat, they could experience vomiting.

I was fortunate that I never felt nausea. Patients who do are often prevented from eating, and that presents a problem—cancer patients need to eat in order to take in the nutrition required to boost their immune systems. A strong immune system is critical when fighting cancer. The only side effect I ever suffered was a mouth that tasted like cardboard and joint pain for a day or two after treatments. Here was the deal I made with nausea: I won't go looking for you if you won't come looking for me. During subsequent treatments I was more discreet when I ate lunch. But I made sure to eat because my primary focus was to ardently advocate for myself—through prayer, meals, vitamins, and the health drink and juicer that were so generously provided to me by the Martin and Villalobos/Garcia families.

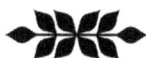

CHAPTER FIFTEEN

Never Missed a Day of Work

My chemo schedule was one treatment a month for the next six months. As I already mentioned, my first session went rather well. As the chemicals flowed through my body, I visualized them as agents that were seeking out and destroying evil cancer cells. In my mind the cancer cells were being attacked and dying off. To put it politely, they were getting their blocks knocked off. Throughout the process I felt empowered by God, who had placed my oncologist in my life.

After several chemo sessions, I discovered that many of the other patients being treated were also educators. That seemed strange to me. Could the disease have been influenced by the environment we found ourselves working in or the stress of the job? Maybe it was a combination of both. Teaching can be challenging to one's health. It's a job that you show up for every day, regardless of how you feel.

I never missed a day of work during my battle with cancer. As a matter of fact, I never missed a day of work ... period. I'm sure my principal and many staff members wondered how I kept my attendance up during this challenging period of time. But I wasn't functioning merely as a physical being; my body was also operating off of *spiritual motivation*. I prayed to God to help me finish out the school year with my students. I do not like to start a job and not finish it. That has been my nature all my life.

One motivating force came from a colleague in our school district whom we all admired. Her name was Debbie. She also battled cancer and never lost a day of work. Eventually, Debbie lost her battle, but her courage earned her tremendous respect from her coworkers. Despite losing her life, Debbie inspired us all to be strong. Among other things, she taught us not to be afraid to ask a cancer patient, "How are you feeling today?" or "How's your day going?" Having Debbie around helped take away the discomfort people felt when interacting with a cancer patient in the workplace. I remember thinking, "How is Debbie able to come to work every day?" After I was stricken with cancer, I discovered the answer: She stood up and fought her cancer. She knew she could not lie down and give up.

Debbie will always be remembered. She lives on in the hearts of those who knew her. She was courageous in her fight and completely dedicated to her students.

Debbie's courageous effort helped increase my energy and motivation to teach my students the way I was committed to teaching them. I made every effort to be the most effective teacher I could be, especially now that I was starting my chemotherapy sessions. My students' efforts were reciprocal. They did the best they could under adverse conditions—knowing that their teacher had cancer. Even though their teacher had thrown them a curveball, they were handling it with great poise. My students were aware of what I was attempting to accomplish: Take one day at a time and give them everything I had until we reached the end of the school year.

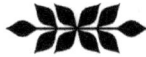

CHAPTER SIXTEEN

The Results Are In

At the end of six months I completed my last chemo session. My oncologist ordered X-rays so we could see what the treatments had accomplished. Despite having lost all my hair, I was feeling pretty good at this stage of the game. I was even putting on weight, which was a positive sign. The weight gain, along with the daily juice recipe provided by Bill and Ernestine Martin, helped me boost my immune system and keep fighting.

At this point I was feeling good physically *and* spiritually. I just *knew* that my tumors had shrunk. If the X-rays showed they had, we would be on the positive side of the scoreboard; we would be winning the fight.

The results came in. With our hearts in our mouths my wife and I waited in my oncologist's office to receive the results. After we heard his enthusiastic knock on the examination room door, my

oncologist entered with X-ray films under his arms.
He said, "I have great news for both of you. There
aren't any noticeable tumors."

At first my wife and I didn't understand what
he was saying. He repeated his statement, "There
aren't any tumors showing up on the X-rays." We
couldn't believe our ears. God had delivered a
miracle into our lives. It's hard to explain how my
wife and I felt. We both shed tears of joy.

My oncologist said, "I am very encouraged with
the results of your chemo treatments. However, I
still would like you to take the radiation treatments
as part of the program that I've planned for you.
But first I would like to schedule a CAT scan to be
sure we've gotten all of the cancer."

My wife and I agreed to his approach. God had
heard all the prayers that had been sent. I had been
blessed. My wife and I were dazed from the excellent news. We couldn't wait to notify everyone who
cheered me on and helped me reach this stage in
my treatments. God was responding to our prayers.

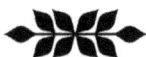

CHAPTER SEVENTEEN
Radiation Treatment

Several weeks later I received my appointment schedule for thirty or more consecutive radiation treatments. I met with a team of radiologists at a private radiology center located in Chula Vista, California. The team of radiologists was very positive; they seemed to carry on where my oncologist and his staff left off with regard to excellent caregiving. The fact that my CAT scan had come back clean created optimism in all of us for a favorable outcome. Praises to God were in order.

Before receiving my first radiation treatment, my chest was charted with permanent markings that directed the radiation during each treatment. Without those marks, they would have had to repeat the charting each visit, and that would have taken a lot of time. As a result of the permanent markings, radiation treatments were a breeze, and I didn't suffer any side effects in the short run. After each treatment, I jumped up from the radiation table, put on my shirt, and headed out to teach my adult school class, which was located a few blocks away. I have had only one radiation side effect over the years: I am unable to lift things that are extremely heavy. This limitation is a small price to pay for good health. The scar tissue in my left chest area reminds me to remain humbled to my God-given miracle.

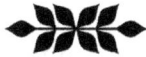

CHAPTER EIGHTEEN

A New Student or an Angel?

Throughout my entire cancer ordeal my students were wonderful—those in my elementary class as well as those in my adult class. One evening I received a new adult student. He had a mild-mannered demeanor that distinguished him from other people I had come in contact with. After about a week of attending my class, he came up to talk with me and mentioned my battle with cancer. Then he asked me how I was coming along. The strangest thing was that I had never mentioned anything about my battle to my adult students, whom I already had been teaching for six months. By the time he approached me, my radiation treatments were behind me, and I was a seasoned warrior in the battle. I rarely thought about being a cancer patient anymore. Instead, I thought of myself as a survivor.

The new student went on to ask, "Would you

mind if I and the Prayer Warriors of my church pray for you?" I was amazed that a stranger would show such sincere concern about my health, especially because I had not discussed it in front of him. "Yes." I replied. "That would be just fine with me." I make it a habit never to turn down a prayer.

Next, this student requested that I write my name down on a piece of paper. I did as he requested and handed the paper to him. I thanked him several times, and I'm glad that I did because after that day I never saw him again.

I refer to this student as an angel because there was something special about his soft-spoken nature. If he was merely a student who didn't return for whatever reason, I would like to thank him for taking my name into prayer with people who didn't even know me. If, on the other hand, he was an angel, it was an absolute pleasure to have communicated directly with a gift-bearer sent from God.

By this time I started to believe that I really was in favor with God, in whom I had placed my trust. You can't imagine how wonderful my wife and I were feeling at this point.

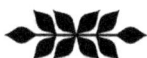

CHAPTER NINETEEN

Never Give Up

Shortly after I had been diagnosed with lung cancer, I learned that my next-door neighbor had been diagnosed with pancreatic cancer. Pancreatic cancer metastasizes at a very rapid pace, which means it spreads cells from one part of the body to another. A very aggressive course of treatment is necessary to fight pancreatic cancer. After some individuals hear they have cancer, any kind of cancer, they give up ... they throw in the towel. Conversely, others start fighting immediately. Staying positive is an important tool; it can increase your chances of winning the battle.

My neighbor was one of those patients who chose to lie down and give up. His attitude disturbed his wife, who on several occasions begged my wife and me to come over and get her husband out of bed. She knew that I was fighting my own battle with cancer, and she saw that our attitudes were different; she saw that I wasn't acting as though anything was wrong with me.

My neighbor and I had been given the same fate: facing death in about three months. We were told that if we were lucky, we might be able to extend that a month or two. However, the difference between my neighbor and me was that I chose to stand up and fight. And I welcomed support in my efforts: God, my oncologist, my wife, myself, my family, my friends, my coworkers, and the angels who appeared along the way. All of these people wrapped their arms around me and helped me to live and flourish.

My wife and I informed my neighbor's wife that we would pray for her husband. Prayer is very important during times of illness; I found the prayers of others to be calming and comforting during my battle with cancer. Even though I thought twice about interjecting religion into my neighbor's situation, I thought my prayer would be welcomed with little hesitation. For those who don't have God in their lives, it's never too late to invite Him into your hearts.

Of course, I understand that believers who pray succumb to illnesses every day. Nevertheless, it is helpful to remember that we did not come here to stay. We are here for a limited duration of time, and we have nothing to lose when we hold out our hands to God. Our final blessing will be to move on into the presence of God.

CHAPTER TWENTY

Stand Up with Dignity

The most important things to do to maintain good health are to stay positive, have faith, and pray. When people hear that God performed a miracle for me after a three-month prognosis, when they hear me say "God saved my life," they feel inspired. They begin to understand that only God can decide when we leave. One day, when God chooses, I will depart. Meanwhile, hopefully it can be said that I have encouraged and motivated people to stand up for themselves.

One evening my wife and I heard a loud knocking on our front door. It was our ill neighbor; he was standing in front of our door as frail as could be. In fact, he was so weak that we almost didn't recognize him. When he had been in good health, he stood at least six feet four inches tall. However, now that he had cancer, that wasn't the case. Our neighbor was bent over, but he was still standing. As he looked at my wife and me, he expressed with his eyes, "I am standing. Do you see me?" His courage that day meant so much to us. Our neighbor was standing … with dignity. I am sure his wife wanted to accompany him to our house; however, this was *his* moment. His wife and family were proud that he had garnered the courage to, literally, stand up to cancer. My wife and I were proud of him, as well.

Our neighbor passed away shortly after that evening. I am sure that he moved on to a better place and that he is with God. My neighbor's wife and family cherish the strength, dignity, and faith their loved one displayed in his final days. As with Debbie, my former colleague, my neighbor will remain in my heart always. He demonstrated inner strength at the very last moment of his life. He taught me that it is never too late to leave a positive impression about who you are at your core … despite debilitating illness.

CHAPTER TWENTY-ONE

Postscript: Cancer Free

It's been over thirteen years since I've been cancer free. My miraculous healing (after a three-months-to-live prognosis) has provided me with the opportunity to encourage many other people to stay positive and fight their cancer *standing up*. Throughout the years I have extended my positive message—to colleagues at the district office or other schools and to family members—and of course, shared my Bill and Ernestine Martin juice recipe with those who needed it.

I know that I've been blessed, and I am humbled when people ask me to tell my story or explain the importance of remaining positive when things appear to be so bleak. I am quick to point out to others who have been stricken with cancer that I have been blessed with a miracle and that God has one waiting for them … if they have the courage to trust, stay positive, and partner with God by taking steps to promote good health. Even though I am aware that each person has his or her own way of embracing spirituality, my primary message is hope.

I hope and pray that those who receive a cancer diagnosis will seek out a higher being who can hear their prayers because that's where miracles come from. Every time I see a sunrise, I am reminded of God's grace, and every time a new attending physician looks up from my chart and says, "Do you know that you are a miracle?" I am filled with love and gratitude. It is often difficult for doctors to believe that I am still alive. When they express their surprise and wonderment, I immediately agree and say, "All praises to God that I am still alive." Sometimes it's difficult to understand the enormity of my many blessings, but one thing is certain: I thank God all day long for the blessings he has bestowed upon me.

I also attribute my blessings to the contributions I have made as a teacher. At one time I planned to practice law, but subsequently, I became deeply affected by the level of influence teachers can have on the lives of children. Teachers live on in the hearts of so many people. We all remember one teacher who inspired us to learn or another teacher who motivated his or her colleagues. Teachers are a very special group of people. It is their responsibility to prepare our students for the future, and if we fail to do so, we have failed ourselves; when we have failed ourselves, we have failed our nation. Pouring myself into my family and profession enabled me to feel like a worthy, contributing member of society—despite my diagnosis.

I thank God for giving me thirteen years beyond my initial plea to finish out the "the new school year." I made good use of that time. I loved family and friends and received their love in return. I dedicated myself to our nation's children, and I gave hope when it seemed all was lost. I am humbled by all I have been able to achieve in my lifetime … thanks to my attitude, my love of God, and my miracle from heaven.

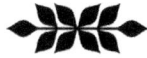

Appendix

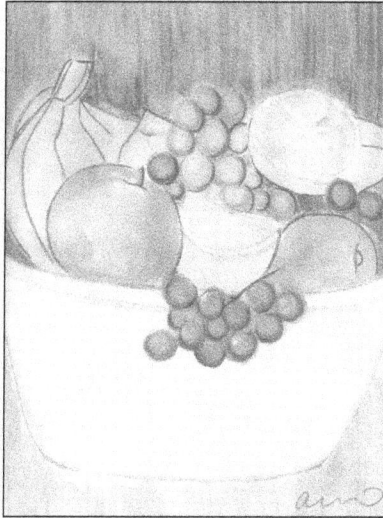

~ Vitamins and Supplements for Health ~
~ Veggies for Health ~
~ Juicer Recipe ~
~ Irungu's Prayer of Gratitude ~
~ Irungu's Prayer for His Readers ~
~ Psalm 30 ~
~ Resources, Books and Information ~

Irungu's Miracle Program

The right doctor with the right attitude

Information: books and Internet

Medical treatment as prescribed by doctors

Juicer recipe

Vitamins and supplements

Immune-building nutrition (lots of veggies)

Visualizations

Work

God

Church

Prayer

Family support

Friends' support

Coworkers' support

Helping others

Positive attitude

Trust in a positive outcome

Vitamins and Supplements for Health

Selenium: is an antioxidant that blocks molecules known as free radicals, which are known to damage DNA. The combination of vitamin C, vitamin E, and selenium may help guard against cancer.

Vitamin C: is an antioxidant that offers protection against cancer.

Vitamin E: protects cellular membranes. It also helps the body use selenium to destroy or neutralize damaging free radicals, thereby lowering the risk of cancer.

Irungu's Supplement Regimen Per Day

Selenium (200 mcg)
Vitamin C (1,000 mg)
Vitamin E (400 iu)

Veggies for Health

Beets: betacyanin (fights tumors and defends cells against harmful carcinogens)

Broccoli: vitamin C, A, and folate

Brussels sprouts: vitamin C, A, E, and iron

Cabbage: vitamin C, potassium, folate, and betacarotene (strengthens the immune system and fortifies cell membranes)

Carrots: vtamin A (betacarotene)

Cauliflower: Vitamin C, B6, folate, and potassium

Celery: Vitamin C

Celery leaves (usually discarded): vitamin A, iron, and potassium

Collard greens: vitamin C, calcium, iron, potassium, bioflavonoids, carotenoids, and other cancer-fighting compounds

Corn: complex carbohydrates and fiber

Kale: Bioflavonoids and carotenoids (cancer-fighting compounds)

Onion family: onions, chives, leeks, scallions, and shallots have powerful phytochemicals and fiber that may protect against cancer

Spinach: Vitamin A and bioflavonoids (help block cancer)

Sweet potatoes: vitamin A (betacarotene), C, and B6

Fruits for Health

Pomegranate: Laboratory studies show that various components of the pomegranate suppress the growth of human breast cancer cells and could reduce the spread of lung cancer. The pomegranate has always been one of my favorite fruits; as a youngster I looked forward to it showing up in stores during the fall season. Because of its antioxidant-rich content, the pomegranate was my number one fruit of choice in my battle against cancer. Historically, the pomegranate has been traced back to ancient Egypt. From there it was spread by the Greeks to the Middle East and to Europe. The pomegranate is mentioned in the *Bible* over two dozen times. It is said to have 613 seeds, a figure that corresponds to the original number of commandments.

Apricots: Betacarotene (antioxidant) protects against the cell damage that occurs when the body burns oxygen, a process that can lead to the development of cancer and other diseases.

Cherries: Contain phytochemicals that may help fight certain cancers.

Grapefruit: High in pectin, a soluble fiber that helps lower blood cholesterol. Pink and red varieties have lycopene, an antioxidant that may lower the risk of prostate cancer.

Melons: Vitamin A, C, potassium, and other minerals. Cantaloupes and other yellow varieties are high in betacarotene, which helps protect against cancer and other diseases.

Oranges: Vitamin C (antioxidant) protects against cell damage by free radicals and may reduce certain cancers. Oranges also contain rutin, hesperidins, and other bioflavonoid plant pigments that also act as antioxidants and may help prevent or retard tumor growth.

Tomatoes: Lycopenes (bioflavonoid) are alleged prostate-cancer-fighting agents.

Juicer Recipe

Irungu drank twice per day.

4 carrots
1 apple
½ beet
4 sprigs parsley
2 stalks celery

Irungu's Prayer of Gratitude

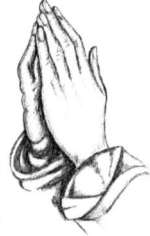

Dear Lord,

I thank you for your many blessings and my
extended gift of life. You have walked with
me, carried me, and at different times let me walk alone
to test my courage to fight against cancer. At other times
you've tested the faith that I had in you. As you know, I
never wavered. I trusted you every inch of the way, to bring
a Miracle into my life.

—AMEN

Irungu's Prayer for His Readers

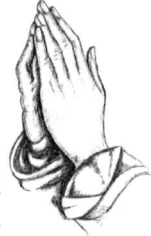

Lord,
Please bless the readers of my book who find
themselves facing their own battles with can-
cer. I pray that they find the courage and faith to receive
the many blessings you have waiting for them. May family
members and friends also find the inspiration to trust and
believe that Miracles do happen each and every day.
—Amen

Psalm 30

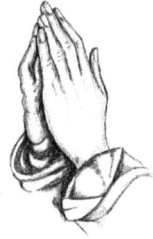

I will exalt you, O Lord,
for you lifted me out of the depths
and did not let my enemies gloat over me.
O Lord, my God,
I called to you for help,
and you healed me.
O Lord, you brought me up from the grave;
you spared me from going down into the pit.

Sing to the Lord, you saints of His,
praise His holy name.
For his anger lasts only a moment,
but his favor lasts a lifetime.
Weeping may remain for a night,
but rejoicing comes in the morning.

When I felt secure,
I said, "I will never be shaken."
O Lord, when you favored me,
you made my mountain stand firm.
But when you hid your face,
I was dismayed.
To you, O Lord, I called;
to the Lord I cried for mercy:
"What gain is there in my destruction,
in my going down into the pit?

Will the dust praise you?
Will it proclaim your faithfulness?
Hear, O Lord, and be merciful to me;
O Lord, be my help."

You turned my wailing into dancing;
you removed my sackcloth and clothed me with joy,
that my heart may sing to you and not be silent.
O Lord, my God, I will give you thanks forever.

Resources, Books and Information

A Cancer Battle Plan
by Anne Fraham & David Fraham

City of Hope at:
www.CityOfHope.org

Cancer Treatment Centers of America at:
www.CancerCenter.com

Mayo Clinic at:
www.MayoClinic.com

Research and Information at:
www.Healthline.com

◆━❈❈━◆

About the Author

Having a tremendous will to survive, Irungu Adeyemi refused to give up; with courageous action steps he partnered with God to defeat the deadly clutches of lung cancer. Irungu's love for his wife, family, and students supplied him the inspiration he needed to live. Irungu's medical miracle motivated him to write an inspirational book to help cancer patients and their family members overcome their fears.

Irungu A. Adeyemi attended Foothill College, Los Altos Hills, California, and the University of California, San Diego, where he earned his B.A. He received his law degree at Western Sierra Law School, San Diego, California. He retired from a teaching career at the National School District and the Regional Occupational Program (Sweetwater Union H.S. District). Irungu is a U.S. Navy veteran of the Cuban Missile Crisis era.

Irungu has inspired his colleagues and others with his message of hope. He challenges all of us to live by a wise, profound navy tradition, "Never let the wind out of your sail when you are faced with uncertainty and adversity."

Having been cancer free for over thirteen years (after receiving a three-month prognosis), Irungu is looking forward to publishing his children's books, which are also filled with inspiration.

Irungu lives in the Temecula Valley of Southern California with his wife, Marilyn. He is lovingly involved with his children and grandchildren who live in Temecula, San Diego, and Philadelphia.

To order more copies of this book, or to find out more about Irungu's current projects, visit:
www.AdeyemiBooks.com